So I'm
A Reiki Practitioner,
What NOW?

All you need to know when you become a Certified Reiki Practitioner

Jackie Ward

GW00459210

Special Thanks

I owe everything to my best friend, my partner in life, my husband - Ian. He is always there, behind the scenes, supporting me in everything I do. Without your continued support and encouragement I would not have had the confidence to be practising Reiki, teaching Reiki or writing this book about Reiki. It is only with your love that I am able to be doing all that I love xx

Important Disclaimer

This book is designed to provide information on ways to move forward after your Reiki Class and practise Reiki on yourself, family, friends or in a professional manner.

It is not the purpose of this book to reprint all the information that is otherwise available to new Reiki Practitioners, but instead to complement, amplify and supplement the learning. You are urged to read all the available material, learn as much as possible about Reiki and interrelated therapies and practices and tailor the information to your individual needs.

The purpose of this book is to educate and entertain. The author shall have neither liability nor responsibility to any person or entity with respect to any loss or damage caused or alleged to have been caused, directly or indirectly, by the information contained in this book.

Table of Contents

About the Author

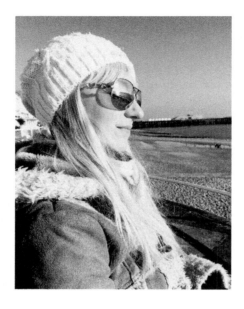

Jackie first discovered Reiki in 1994 and is now a practising and teaching Reiki Master, who devotes her spare time to encouraging new practitioners, answering their questions and providing emotional and practical support through various media.

Jackie previously worked as a Nurse before meeting her husband, starting their family and home-schooling their 2 children for 9 years. She learnt Reiki along the way, first coming across it during her nurse training in 1996 whilst working on a very challenging Cancer Ward in London. She soon found it to be the tool she was looking for to help her with her own relaxation, stress and any physical ailments. This then extended out to her family and it wasn't long before her love of Reiki extended to her mother and step-father who both went on to become practising and teaching Reiki Masters themselves!

Working from home on a very part-time basis, around the children's upbringing and education; she invested in a second hand Reiki bed and set it up in a tiny little dark, windowless, 'broom cupboard' of a room that had been used for storage. Friends and family healing sessions soon extended to the paying public and she realised that this was something she wanted to do more of and also teach. Teaching sessions and Reiki Shares began to regularly spill over into the family living room.

She now continues to practise Reiki alongside EFT and Matrix Reimprinting both in person and online at www.stleonardsreiki.co.uk
Jackie teaches all levels of Reiki, from her now much larger and brighter Treatment Room, in

St Leonards on Sea on the South Coast of England. It is during this teaching and in her monthly Reiki Shares that the many questions and answers have been raised and she now wants to extend this information to as many new practitioners of Reiki as possible, via this book.

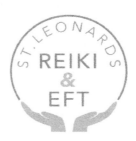

www.stleonardsreiki.co.uk

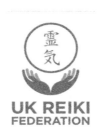

Introduction

So I am guessing that you have your Reiki 1 Certificate proudly framed at home. You loved it so much and decided to make the leap to the Reiki 2 Practitioner Level. Now having just completed your Reiki 2 Course/Workshop, it may seem as though everything has changed in your outlook of the world and you feel that you now need to adjust and make changes in your life. You may have actually allowed yourself to believe that you can be a Reiki Practitioner and ordered your business cards and even bought your insurance! You have changed so much as a person and really have no idea what your next step is. Well, this is where I imagine you may be if you are reading this? Once upon a time, I was in that very same position.

I could see that other people were running a successful Reiki business but even after my wonderful training and the many supportive words from my Reiki Master, I was eventually left to my own devices and alone with my Certificates and what seemed like just dreams.

Completing a Reiki course isn't like passing other regular activities, like your driving test or A-Levels. No-one really wants to talk to you about it, least of all family and friends. The subject is changed as quickly as the mention of Reiki is raised. Other than those other lovely like-minded souls on your Course, there really is a sense of alienation and impossibility.

Well that was my story anyway. I say this to assure you that I've made all the mistakes possible in setting up a Reiki business. In fact, it is only now that I have completely immersed myself in the world of teaching, that I realise how important it is for me to share my failings and insecurities, in the hope that I can save just one of you from some of the stumbling blocks I encountered along the way.

So Now I'm A Practitioner - Help!

Learning Reiki is quite a game changer isn't it?
Whether it was a group you trained in, as a one-to-one,
a day, or a weekly course....they are more of a life
journey than a course. Often really getting you doing
some soul searching and re-evaluating everything you
thought you knew about yourself, your upbringing and
your whole outlook on the Universe.

Wherever it was you were when you began your Reiki
learning, I can guarantee everything feels different
now. Am I right? You found a like-minded soul in
your Reiki Master, who walked you through your
learning and you may have made some real
connections with others in the class. Amongst the
support, essential oils, crystals, candles and soft music
you felt so comfortable in, you now find yourself back
in reality with all its restrictions, limitations,
expectations and duties. Whatever is next?

The following chapters are some of the fleeting
thoughts and experiences that may resonate with you
at this moment in time. To just know that you are not
alone right now, is important and to realise that there is
a path along which you can tread, which is neither mad
nor insane; but achievable and realistic.
Please dip into this book as you need. Some if not all of
it may be relevant to you now. Both professional
advice is outlined as well as some self-care tips for your
personal health and wellbeing during this time of
change and adjustment.

Why Does Everything Seem So Different Now?

Reiki is not about healing as much as it is a journey to the center of the Universe - Ourselves!

It's like you've outgrown your body and see everything differently all of a sudden. Why does this happen?

Well, you have to start with yourself before you can help anyone else. You need to be in the best place possible before you have the room and space to assist others. It's all good, all part of the healing process. You are just adjusting to the new energy and coming back to self. We kind of get a bit lost in life and forget where we are going and who we are. Quite often, a Reiki Course can leave you questioning everything but also re-assessing exactly what it is that's important to you and where it is you want to go, but never realised before. Celebrate all these emotions, they are fleeting. You might be feeling a little uncomfortable but it truly is a cause for celebration - it means that you are awake and more alive than ever! You have just poked your head out from the fog.

Obviously, we are not just talking about a day course, to have this affect on you, this may be way way down the line, after your course, after many months of self treatment, further reading, contemplation and finally, FINALLY actually being able to meditate for more than 5 minutes at a time.

Why Do My Friends and Family Not Understand Me and All That I'm Going Through?

Yes, people around you may be thrilled for you that you seem happier. However, if this 'change' in you means that the people around you are now expected to make changes in lifestyle that affects them, they may quite rudely scoff at anything you then suggest and become a little defensive.

This is a biggy and and can have a real impact on relationships. We often start a Reiki Course in one place and finish in a completely different place to where we began. (We are talking emotionally, not locations) This 'shift' is hard enough for us to adjust to. So is it really that hard for us to expect our loved ones to understand? Bless them, they're still there, where we left them, wondering who this new person is that's come home to them. Now don't get me wrong, this new found confidence and sense of self is often celebrated and very well received and partners have come along soon after to find out what it is their loved ones have found and they are missing out on. However, this is not always the case and difficulties can and do arise.

Understand that all that's happened is that you have changed your personal outlook a little. Probably undone some of your long standing fears and don't feel so restricted anymore. More things seem possible now, even natural and you are ready to move forward in a direction you never would have dreamt about before. Just realise and respect that the people around you are still standing in your old shoes.

You're keen to share this new amazing skill you've just learnt. You're doing your daily self treatment and really benefiting from it and loving it. Maybe you are lucky enough to have a pet or two that is allowing you to give them Reiki. However, you are literally desperate to get your hands on someone. (In a healing capacity) You either can't convince your loved ones to be your guinea pig or they are giving you such negative vibes, you daren't even go there! All I will say is that if people around you are not immediately receptive to receiving a Reiki Treatment, don't push it!! We should never force Reiki on anyone :-) In fact, I often suggest to my students that they do quite the opposite.

A change in your energy, affects the energy both within and around you and the perceptive around you, will pick up and notice this immediately. You may be met by people and told that you look lighter or have a radiance or a glow about you. People will be intrigued and want to find out more.

So my philosophy is to let people pull it out of you to the point of begging you for a Reiki Treatment. Not vice versa!

There should always be an energy exchange even in these early days. A trade for your services, either money, cake or a favour. Yes I understand that you're desperate to practise and the payment isn't important, but it is always necessary for an effective treatment. As you have been taught, mankind has a fascination for money and nothing given away or offered voluntarily, unfortunately, holds any worth in many people's minds.

Trade is a great place to start and swaps are a wonderful idea. Practitioners are generally lousy at looking after themselves, much like a decorator living in an undecorated house all their life. So when you meet and treat a reflexologist, massage therapist or beautician, etc. suggest you keep in touch and swap therapies and it's a win win for you both.

Practise Self Care!

Slowly Does It. Understand that you are going through changes and that this may result in a variety of emotions surfacing. In this chapter, I outline a few ways you can help yourself during this transitional period of your life.

Fear

This is number one! I remember feeling really frustrated, not understanding how to make the changes necessary to work as a Reiki Practitioner and where on earth to begin? The amazing spiritual high felt at the end of the Reiki training is very often, physically unsustainable. Be patient and forgiving with yourself. All the while you strive to move forward, there will naturally be resistance lurking in your subconscious and as daft as it sounds, quite often you may actually be your worst enemy in moving forward. Just know that it is your fear talking. That part of you that holds us back and prevents us from taking risks in case we hurt ourselves or make a fool of ourselves. Humans are resistant and fearful of change. We prefer the safety of what we know and most of us like familiarity and the comfort of routine. Phrases like "better the devil you know" will spring to mind.

Your positivity and support networks and continued focus each day, will get you through this initial fearful phase. As you march forward with your goals and plans and surround yourself with like minded people, the fears will diminish and your future path will seem clearer and within reach. Attend Reiki Shares as often as possible. Keep in touch with your Reiki Master and maybe the colleagues you learnt with and continue to read and learn and grow in the direction you are wanting to move into.

If the people around you seem negative towards your new ideas and wishes for the future, don't be angry with them. Remember they are still where you left them before you did your Reiki training. Nothing has changed for them and they can't understand what it is you're banging on about and really are not at all interested. They probably wish you'd never done this Reiki training and hope you soon get back to being your old self again. So send them love not hostility. Remember, it's you who has changed and it doesn't give you the right to take it upon yourself to go about trying to change everyone around you. Your number one priority and purpose in life, is looking after yourself; your energy, your wellbeing and maintaining your emotional and physical balance and harmony. Enjoy continuing to learn about energy and in learning how to understand how to maintain your balance whilst interacting with other people. Don't give yourself a hard time.

Forgiveness

Practise forgiveness both for yourself and others. Recognise that everyone and everything that presents itself to you is a blessing and maybe there is something to learn from if you look hard enough. Acknowledge and respect it/them, then practise forgiveness.

Practising forgiveness is key to moving forward and finding your internal peace and happiness. We often beat ourselves up about mistakes we have made along the way, things we have said and actions we have taken. The road is long and sometimes painful, but we have to take the journey and suffer along the way a little perhaps, in order to find our peace. However, we don't realise that the journey is really all there is. After all, life is not so much just about the end result. It is the struggle that defines us, and the lessons learnt along the way. Living in this moment now is what we need to do, rather than constantly wishing and wanting more and to be somewhere else.

What I am trying to say is that, it is wasted energy, regretting and wishing upon our past mistakes. Our past and all the decisions and actions taken upon our journey, define us and the end result is always the here and now. If you are happy with the here and now, you have reason to celebrate all that has been. You are not the same person you were when you were born, or when you were a teenager. We literally are different versions of ourselves as we grow.

It is obvious that the younger, less experienced version of yourself, would clearly have acted differently compared to the older wiser version of yourself today.

Shame, guilt, remorse…. These are emotions that define you as a human. We all carry varying shades of all emotions. The fact that you feel them, proves that you have grown and learnt from life experience. It does not mean that you should allow yourself to wallow in self pity or suffer eternally because you are consumed with embarrassment of how you have acted in the past. You have been many different versions of yourself and are now trying to be the new brightest, shiniest version yet.

Practising forgiveness releases not only yourself but anyone you feel has wronged you or you have wronged in the past. The act of sending or writing down a statement of forgiveness has tremendous power. A simple thought then made manifest into spoken or written words is then released out into the universe, out into the various fields of energy, becoming a reality and having a ripple effect on everyone and everything around you. Everything is energy.

You don't even have to believe what you say because the act of saying or writing a positive affirmation or statement, changes your energy as you express yourself. If you express this new positive affirmation (never negative), after a time, your initial belief will change and eventually the affirmation will no longer be necessary for you to say, as it will be so. The people you are forgiving or asking forgiveness from, will feel this in their energy and it will have an affect on them also.

Gratitude

Make gratitude your best friend. I know it sounds a bit woo woo; but it's powerful, simple and just works! Form a practise or a mantra, be it writing or speaking, praying, meditating,…. but do it in some way each day and it will transport you into a more loving appreciative, patient person. Soon everything around you and every word that is spoken to you, every song on the radio, will all start to have a personal meaning. You will realise that life certainly is supporting you and speaking to you in every moment at all times in all ways. But first you have to notice these signs and the practise of gratitude is a stepping stone to this place or realisation.

Know that anything that upsets you or brings a rise in your emotions, is important to look at. Why did it cause a reaction within you?

Sometimes it is good to reflect, look at and learn and other times, it is best simply to acknowledge words or actions and then let them float away like a cloud - not allowing the words or actions to upset us and unbalance us, but just simply move on.

When you realise that others are often simply projecting their own internal fears and insecurities outwardly, it makes it easier to be unaffected. When you understand that often others' words or actions are not actually personal to you in any way just because they were directed at you, it is easier to maintain your energy. You begin to realise that expression is often just an outpouring of emotional energy that needed releasing and you just happened to get the brunt of it. This realisation, then releases you from making everything so personal and actually allows you to be more grateful for yours and others outward expression.

Your voice is your greatest manifesting tool. Singing, poetry, laughing, crying, writing, journalling, story telling…….. are all forms of healthy expression and should be celebrated. Emotions held within, fester and yearn for release. A blocked throat chakra is often a sign that difficulties around communication are causing either emotional or physical problems.

The simple act of practising gratitude can change your energy immediately. It can awaken you and focus you in what is all around you but that you may have taken for granted.

Quite often we have all we need right there in front of us. We are constantly searching outwardly for happiness, but often in the wrong places. Happiness lies within.

Start with practising gratitude for all that you have to begin with and then you can move forward and work with practising gratitude to bring about and manifest all that you desire and need.

Drink Water

After your Attunement, there will be shifts in your energy. Your Reiki Master I am sure, would have encouraged you to look after yourself and hopefully during your 21 Day Cleanse, you gave yourself plenty of self Reiki and drank plenty of water. I need to express the importance of drinking plenty of water. rinking enough fluid is just another part of self care. Your body is your temple and is approximately 60% water. Without it you would not live for long. It is amongst the main ingredients for life. Water breeds life.

Water is important not just to drink but has a huge impact on our emotional well being. Water balances, soothes and promotes our sense of well being both mentally and physically. If you are not a big water drinker, find a herbal, fruit or ice tea that you enjoy. Or add fruit to a flask of water and make your own infusion. Many illnesses and disease can be exacerbated by a lack of fluid and many people have regular minor health problems due to not taking in enough fluid throughout each and every day, eventually causing long term problems.

I talk about it here, because it is especially important for a Reiki Practitioner to look after themselves after an Attunement when the energy in your body is adjusting to the new vibrations it is aligning itself to.

It makes sense to help your body along, whilst it is adjusting to changes. Sip slowly throughout the day. The average sedentary adult will require 2 - 2.5% litres of fluids in a 24 hour period. This varies depending on weight and lifestyle. Obviously it goes without saying, but I'll say it anyway, that anything in excess can cause problems, so again, it's all about balance.

Stretch

Wake up and stretch. Stretch in between giving Reiki Treatments. Stretch after Reiki Treatments. Stretch at the end of the day. Our body is at its best when it's balanced, inwardly and out.

Through no fault of our own, we have dominant arms and legs which cause our body to compensate in everything we do on a daily basis. Exercise will keep you flexible and supple and able to live in a freer, happier body.

The Healing Crisis

This is talked about more so after a Reiki Treatment and with regards our clients, but we must be aware that a healing crisis can occur for us, the Reiki Practitioners at any time and especially so after the Attunement.

On the physical side, be happy with small aches and pains, whatever they may be. They are a sign that your body is making adjustments for the better. Drinking water and being kind to yourself and giving yourself plenty of self Reiki will all help ease these niggles.

Reiki does not understand or recognise excess medication in the body and will potentially see this as a foreign body and want to release it. Any areas of weakness or where Reiki comes across blockages are most commonly the places, that suffer. Feelings of fatigue, nausea, feeling as though you are coming down with a cold, or an upset tummy, are all common after Attunements.

Emotionally you may feel real changes after your Reiki Course and Attunement. You may just see life differently and find it difficult to adjust to how things were before. I have experienced people who have almost instantly stopped smoking, or drinking alcohol, as they felt that they just didn't need to anymore.

Physically, changes can also happen quickly and I am aware of people's lifelong medication needing to be adjusted and lowered by half after Attunement. There have also been a number of people I have trained that on completing their course, they have made major life changes in their personal lives sometimes realising that some of their friends and loved ones are not in alignment with them any longer. I'm not saying that this is normal and will happen to you! But we all know that sometimes, it just takes a holiday or a break from the norm to gain an insight into your life and a Reiki Course, can certainly do this!

Making Reiki A Habit

The most important step you can take is to make energy therapy a part of your daily routine. If you want to change even the tiniest part of your world, you need to take care of the carer.

It all starts with you. I always say to students that my classes are just the start. The practise they then go off and the experience they then gain in their daily self Reiki and giving of treatments to friends, family and clients, is where the journey begins.

To experience energy therapy is completely unique for each individual and has to be practised to learn from. There really are parts to Reiki that cannot be taught as such.

The basics are to embrace it in every part of your day and make it a life choice.

*   Upon waking, practise Gratitude, realising all you have to be grateful for, be it your partner, your children, the bed you slept in, the water in the taps, the roof above your head, the view out the window……….

*   Before getting up, practise your Self Reiki, concentrating on any specific areas or just a general overall treatment.

*   Go through your day, being kind to yourself, no negative self talk, interacting with others in a similar vein.

*   Be aware of your energy levels throughout the day. Don't allow others to steal your energy or let it leak out carelessly.

*   Eat little and often. Drink plenty, sipping throughout the day.

*   Notice your intuitive thoughts - don't dismiss them. There is no such thing as coincidence. Begin to listen more to them and allow them and respect them.

*   Listen to your physical body. Let it talk to you and notice the whispers.   Don't wait until it then has to shout and scream to get your attention.

*   Exercise gently every day - activities such as gardening and walking count! We need to be active, it is good for body and mind. Physical activities allow us to be expressive and creative during which time our minds quieten.

*   Allow yourself treats often, lazy baths with scented candles, an hour on the sofa curled up with your favourite book, listening to music …

*   Begin to trust in who you are and who you are becoming and like and embrace it all!

*   Nap in the day if you need to, if your sleep was interrupted in the night.

*   Try to retire to bed at about the same time each night and wake at the same time each morning. Our bodies like discipline and routine.

*   Read in bed in the evening, to tire your eyes and this gives the left side of your brain time to wind down rather than stimulating it as does time spent looking at screens.

*   Try to get 8 hours of sleep each night. There is so much that happens during this time, so we need to make sure this is a big priority. Reiki is primarily about relaxation and allowing that space for the body to be in the optimum state for it to do as it does naturally; balance, energise and heal. This is all happening each night during sleep, but if we are constantly sleep deficient, we will begin to feel unwell and prone to illness and disease due to a weakening immune system and an inability to function effectively, physically and mentally, which will then impact on our emotional well being.

*   If upon waking in the night, you have difficulty getting back off to sleep again, go through the Reiki Self treatment hand positions. This works beautifully, like counting sheep for the mind and you will soon drift off. Spend some time sending distant Reiki to a friend or family member using the visualisation technique. I don't think this has ever failed in helping me fall back into a deep sleep in no time. The left side of our brain is always needing something to do. It's like giving the demanding child a new toy to play with.

Distant Reiki For Self First

Upon first learning Reiki, you should always start with yourself before extending what you have learnt to others. There is a natural progression and order in learning Reiki. The First Level introduced you to self treatment. Reiki 2 is still about you! After your Reiki 2 classes, you should be armed with all the tools to be able to effectively send Reiki to your own past and future. So before diving in and offering to send Reiki to all your relatives around the world, spend some time practising, honing your skill and send Reiki primarily to yourself.

You're a Time Traveller Now

I think this part of Reiki is neglected and I don't know why because it is SO effective and powerful. Maybe people just speak less about it. Personally, I have worked a lot on my own past and visited memories from the past where emotionally or physically I felt I would benefit from Reiki. I find that upon re-visiting episodes of your life from the past, the mixture of actively sending oneself Reiki and observing from a safe distance, is a remarkably effective therapeutic tool. I can't deny that it can be emotional but it is often through these tears that shifts of energy are released and a realisation reached that was not there before, thus creating a new found freedom that may otherwise have been unattainable.

Following my Reiki 2 Practitioner learning, many years later, when learning Matrix Reimprinting, I felt this to be a very similar process, and an almost natural progression from the distant reiki work I had been doing on myself.

I strongly believe that a regular self practise of distant reiki can really bring about balance and harmony within self at a very deep level.

Incorporate your self distant healing and self treatment regime into a regular practise and you should be well on your way to seeing or feeling some real benefits. I'm sure if you don't notice immediately, there will be those around you who will. It may be the odd comment like, "you look so much lighter", "you are glowing" and you will wonder what they are talking about and presume it's your new hairdo or outfit; but it may well be that they are seeing a change in your energy and the energy that surrounds you.

Don't let a lifetime spent believing things have to be hard work for little benefit. This is certainly not always the case. Reiki is joyfully simplistic and easy and with regular practise, gives a massive return. Oh and by the way, it's free therapy for yourself forever!

I Want To Become A Reiki Practitioner, but Where On Earth Do I Start?

It is healthy and in our nature and at the core of our very being to need to create, move on, have dreams and wishes and want to pursue goals and desires. It is only natural after learning and being full of excitement, to then want to share this with others and do what it is you love doing, on a regular basis. Wouldn't it be incredible to do something you love doing and make a living doing it! Well hold on to your hats guys because trust me, this is definitely a reality for you if you are serious and motivated.

Maybe you have literally just woken up and decided that this is what you now want to do, or perhaps the idea has been lurking and creeping up on you very slowly over many years. So
let's talk now about putting the wheels in motion.

Everything that is in existence now, once started out as a thought in somebody's head. So, just know that you are on the right track! However it's all good and well thinking about something and may be all some people do for their entire lives, but to make this thought become a reality, you need to then move this thought state onwards. This is initially done in a variety of simple ways. I believe there are literally 8 steps to achieve your dreams.

*   The Power of Positivity
*   Visualisation

* Using Affirmations with Your Reiki Box
* Gratitude (again!)
* Meditation
* Planning and Goal Setting Using A Vision Board
* Journalling
* Chakra Work and Heart Chakra Meditation

The Power of Positivity

The thoughts we have on a daily basis are generally the same day-in, day-out and when you stop to realise that we have about 60,000 - 80,000 thoughts a day, that is quite scary, especially if they are often negative! So the first place to start is in your mind and to monitor your thoughts.

Try to eliminate any negativity and replace it with positivity. It is surprising when we are observing ourselves, how awful we are to ourself; we really are our own worst enemies. Constantly putting ourselves down and expressing our limited abilities. Notice this now and adapt as quickly as possible. It is just a learnt behaviour that can be easily adapted over a short time.

Don't allow yourself to put yourself down. Start to be able to make regular positive statements about yourself to yourself. Perhaps in the mirror whilst washing and getting ready for the day and again in the evening before bed whilst brushing your teeth. This will not be easy at first as we have been programmed for a long time with this negative self talk and it becomes a habit.

The power of the mind can translate whatever is in our thoughts and materialise them into reality. If you focus on doom and gloom and lack, you will remain under that cloud and see and attract nothing else. If you focus on abundance and possibility, you will only see opportunity and potential. We are literally living batteries, attracting and repelling whatever vibration it is we are emitting and therefore receiving.

Each cell in your body emits 1.4 volts of electricity. There are 50 trillion cells in your body, so that's approximately 70 trillion volts of electricity in your body RIGHT NOW. So start to become consciously aware of this and with focus, this energy called 'chi' can be pretty powerful!

Visualisation

Before you can do it, you've got to see it and feel it. Visualisation is a powerful tool to work with and has been documented well in books and films like "The Secret," that explain how the Law of Attraction works.

Remember, we are like walking magnets, without realising it. Our external outer world simply becomes a reflection of our internal world. You really are where you have chosen to be at any given moment: your world is a product of your creation. Now this may seem unfair and I don't mean to offend anyone but it is a reality that we have made many, many decisions along the way and taken many steps to get to where we are now and have had a lot of free will whilst making many of these decisions. It is simply a case of realising this and making many more changes now if you are not where you wish to be any longer.

If we only learnt as children and understood that we are these incredible creative machines with this ability to constantly programme and attract and manifest. As children, we used to daydream and use our imagination on a daily basis. Children often get told off for being in daydream land. This ability to be somewhere else is instinctive and natural to us, we just forget as we get older.

The first step is to embrace with every cell in your being, a picture or vision, in your mind's eye of where it is you would like to now be, or what it is you would like to now be doing. *It needs to be realistic*, otherwise this new vision of yourself is going to continue to just be a dream. So maybe it's seeing yourself leaving your job and having a change in career as a full time Reiki Therapist. Perhaps you envisage yourself working in your own Treatment Room at home, alongside your family, or in a beauty salon or health center. Maybe you would like to incorporate what you are doing already but run Reiki alongside it. Perhaps you need to attend a college, workshop or course and learn other strings to your bow. Maybe you see yourself moving to Ibiza and setting up a retreat. The world really is your oyster and you are only limited by your imagination.

The practise of visualisation is simple. Be specific, and make it as real as possible in your mind. Really believe it. Fill in all the detail using your senses, so that you can taste, smell and feel what it is you are seeing in this blissful moment.

Find the time each day for this visualisation practise. Do it as often as possible and for as long as possible each time. If it helps, put on some soft music and a scented candle and turn the lights down to aid relaxation. Alternatively ask nature to assist and go and sit outside in the sun, or in a nice gentle breeze and close your eyes and enjoy.

In doing this, you are starting the process of drawing to you what it is you wish for. It is just one of the first steps, but don't be flippant, this is powerful stuff and be careful what you wish for! As time goes by, your dream will start to become clearer each time. Each day, you will feel a little closer to this new reality and it will begin to not feel so out of reach. It will start to become familiar like an old friend.

Without realising it, you are creating a shift in your energy and this will slowly (or sometimes quickly!) have a ripple effect on the electro magnetic energy fields of everything and everyone around you. Paired with your new found positivity it is powerful stuff and I promise you that this works. Before long you will start to see signs of some sort, to show you that you are making powerful changes. Just be open to all this possibility and do be careful what you wish for!

Visualise, visualise, visualise. You've got to see it to believe it.

Using Affirmations with Your Reiki Box

Hopefully you learnt about the value of having a Reiki Box during your Reiki 2 Teaching. A Reiki Box is a great way to send distant Reiki to multiple people at the same time, including your own personal goals and ambitions for yourself.

I also hope that you learnt about affirmations and how they can be used with Reiki. An affirmation is a positive statement (containing no negatives at all) used to aid and improve emotional and mental wellbeing. Affirmations are fantastic to use with Reiki and can also be used with clients during a treatment. I regularly write out affirmations for myself, my family and friends and pop them into my Reiki Box. Crystals and photographs can also go in with them and whenever you have a moment, Reiki can be given to the Reiki Box with the intention that the affirmations contained within are all to receive Reiki.
Every now and again, have a sift through and it is wonderful realising how many of them have been achieved and accomplished and you can discard them with great satisfaction.

The visualisations you have been practising can now be written down into various affirmations. This is powerful in many ways, as the act of writing your desires down on paper and getting these thoughts out of your head and in a visible format is a great form of creation in itself. You are a creative machine and this that was once purely thought, now becomes reality as it is spoken or written.

Examples of relevant Affirmations are …….

"Thank you for a regular succession of full-paying clients."

"My Reiki business is busy, successful and growing."

"I am great at what I do. I'm working hard and word is getting out."

"People are needing this service and I can happily provide."

"I can earn a living and support my family by doing what I love!"

"Thank you for the perfect Treatment Room."
"There is a need for more healers in this world."

These may seem a stretch of the imagination at present and I understand that. I can almost hear a few of you chuckling out loud. Please, however, take my advice and understand that the more you move into this realm of possibility, and allow yourself to step into this place you never dreamed possible - signs will appear, doors will begin to open and the dream and reality will begin to merge and overlap. It will happen slowly; but if you truly desire and work hard at what you wish for, it will begin to happen!

Gratitude

Gratitude is such an important topic, it deserves to be mentioned twice. We have touched on the importance of gratitude generally but I want to talk here about the relevance it plays in setting goals for the future.

Alongside the positivity, visualising and affirmations, try to create a constant feeling of gratitude throughout your day. You now need to get more specific and incorporate gratitude with your affirmations and daily life.

Be thankful for what you are drawing toward you. Be thankful for all that it is you are yearning for, as though it is already here. Be thankful for all that you desire and it shall be yours. Notice a couple of the Affirmation examples started with "Thank you for ......" Act and speak as though you are already in the place you see yourself. As said previously, all that is externally, is a reflection of what is and has been internally.

Don't confuse wishing for gratitude! Take care that you are not wishing for any length of time: for wishing is an act in itself - wishing. This state of wishing is then all you will get in return. The Universe is giving you what it is you ask, just more wishing. Alternatively, if you practice gratitude for any length of time, you will create whatever it is you are grateful for.

So start to practice Gratitude for everything that you want to attract as though you already have it, instead of wishing you had it. Trust me, this practise is a game changer!

Meditation

Everything can be gained from meditation. I seem to find myself recommending this to most of my clients in between our Reiki visits. We are all needing a regular time out in this fast and furious world, which seems to take everything from us leaving us feeling depleted and lost.

If you are reading this and wish to work as a Reiki Practitioner, in whatever format, please, please, I urge you please, just do it. People need places and people to go to where they can unwind, and find their balance and calm, now more than ever! Mental health is on the increase with all the pressures from modern day society. Children are stressed from a young age and it seems the innocence and childhood is so short and limited now.

Meditation is hard for us to do. It is not easy. Fact. It is something everyone needs to be doing however. Reiki is easy both to learn and practise and will benefit people as much as meditation. We need to provide Reiki to be easily accessible for as many people to reach. This is fantastic news for new Reiki Practitioners to hear, as there really has never been more need for you!

On a personal note, I use meditation myself in assisting me in drawing new clients to my practise and creating the business I want. You too can do this, it is quite simple. We will talk about meditating and chakras later in this book as it is a great tip to use meditation with chakra work.

Just get yourself into the habit of finding a quiet time and space to sit and be. Play music of your choice and use a mantra if this helps you to focus or simply concentrate on your breath. Don't worry that thoughts keep popping into your head, they will, that's normal; the main thing is that you allow these thoughts to come and then go. Like watching the clouds passing by - you observe in a detached manner, without frustration that anything else is going to happen. You are simply creating a space to just be for a moment.

Just know that all the while you are running around in the world busily DOING stuff; meditation allows you an escape from the doing as you enter the blissful world of creativity and joy. Meditation creates the space that allows you to hear, listen and tap into the Universe and all that it is trying to say to you. You will grow and develop the intuitive part of you that at Reiki 2 has been awakened to amplify this connection with others and the Universe.

You need to go within or you go without.

Planning and Goal Setting Using a Vision Board

Every day, work towards your new future. You can do this by working your way backwards. See where you want to be in your visualisations and meditations and then backtrack. A powerful way to start and great way of manifesting, is to make a vision board. They are wonderful positive visual tools to aid focus and clarity.

Simply cut out pictures, stick photos and positive words and affirmations, on a piece of thick card or board. Really invest some time on a rainy Sunday afternoon perhaps, creating an inspiring vision of your future reality. You could cut out an image of your perfect idyllic treatment room, property to work from, colour schemes, crystals, therapy beds .... Get every detail in and look at it from every angle. Then when your work of art is complete, you need to be brave and hang it, or frame it, in a visible place, where you can and will see it often.

This is another big statement you are making and again will help draw your dreams even closer. Just like the Reiki box goals, only remove or take it down when the picture and goals have been achieved.

Journalling

Again, this is a very good way of getting those thoughts out of your head and consolidating them. When feelings, emotions and thoughts are all whizzing around, it just feels messy and confusing and can make you feel scattered and overwhelmed. By getting them out of your head and onto paper is just a way of processing and creating some order in the chaos.

Pros and Cons lists are wonderful for working out your options. Diaries are a very therapeutic journey for the soul. Journalling is very popular at the moment because it is in between a diary and a vision board. You can get really creative with journalling and alongside your thoughts and notes, include sketches and stick photos and clip inspirational quotes in etc .... Basically it is your positive thoughts and ideas in a beautiful notebook. You probably did this as a child - maybe at school, in the form of scrapbooks. Kind of like a scrapbook for adults. (A bit like those adult colouring books that are also very popular now and also very brilliant.) They can start very simply but then after many hours of time spent with them, soon become a labour of love and very precious especially over time as one realises the power of them. Again, I often find myself recommending doing this to a lot of clients I work with.

Addictive and powerful manifestation tools.

Chakra Work

Chakras are a big part of my Reiki work. I know that not every Reiki Practitioner works with them with their clients but having an awareness of them and understanding how to work with them is helpful not just with clients but also for ourselves. With regards how to propel yourself forward to where you wish to be, working with your chakras can really assist you.

In case, you have not been taught about the 7 main chakras within and around the body, they are basically as follows:-

Root Chakra	Red	Tailbone Survival
Sacral Chakra	Orange	Pelvis Emotions
Solar Plexus Chakra	Yellow	Abdomen Actions
Heart Chakra	Green	Centre of Chest Love
Throat Chakra	Blue	Throat Communication
Brow Chakra	Indigo	Third Eye Intuition
Crown Chakra	Violet	Top of Head Understanding

They are the doorways that allow the Universal Life Force Energy to flow smoothly in and out of the body and throughout the body. Knowing their location, colour and job, enables us to have a greater understanding of ours and other people's energies.

With regards ourselves and our future goals, we can work with our chakras whilst meditating and open ourselves up to being in the best place possible to receiving and sending out the most positive intentions.

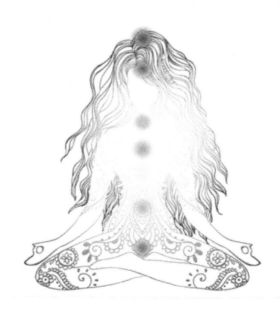

Heart Chakra Meditation

As I said earlier using meditation with chakra work is a powerful manifestation tool. This is a simple heart chakra exercise that I learnt from one of my students. I often use it and would like to share it with you.

When working with the heart chakra, bring your hands to the heart centre and focus on this area. Visualise this green and sometimes pink chakra spinning and strong within your heart centre. Now visualise this chakra rising in the air above you, expanding out all around you bigger and brighter and stronger. Let it rise like a balloon hovering over you and then up into the sky above for all to see. See it shining in the sky like a beacon up there for everyone to recognise and take note. Ask for whoever it is that you are wanting to work with to see your energy there and be drawn to you. You may be above your street, home town, a big city or even the world. Make sure you see the chakra spinning as that gives it its energy and creates momentum. The spinning is pulling the energy into the fields of energy all about you. You are sending out a powerful vibration and the energy you are feeling in this moment will ripple out throughout the energy fields all around you and beyond in all directions.

This is a beautiful and enjoyable meditation to practise and you have my word for it that it works.

Obviously just by doing the above exercise is not enough to attract business solely on its own. You need to be visible for people to find you in the first place, such as notices, advertisements and websites.

Once you have told people you are there, they will then be drawn to you and many will not know why. Put the wheels in motion, do the work and see the results.

A similar exercise can be done with the Solar Plexus Chakra once you are established.

Practise, Practise, Practise

There's no doubt about it, practise makes perfect. There's nothing better than getting out there and doing it. If this is what you are wanting to do, then do it. Even if there are no customers - yet, start practising. It isn't a great idea to push Reiki upon people, but you can certainly offer your services to all and sundry. Nursing homes, care homes, rest homes, hospitals, voluntary organisations, charities, are all excellent places to start. Explain that you are building up your practice and are wanting to increase your experience by offering Reiki on a voluntary basis. Quite often there will be an exchange of some sort, such as food and drink, but voluntary work often leads to paid work.

Word of mouth is the best form of advertising and if you are vocal and participating in your community, you will be seen and heard. Make sure that the people you are working with know all about the business you are working towards so always have a ready supply of business cards or flyers advertising your services to hand.

Fairs and Health and Wellbeing Events are very popular and there should be one local to you that you could attend. To have a stand simply involves offering Reiki for a small charge as a taster to as many people as possible. They get to try a treatment and meet you and you get to network and spread the word, again being visible and out there for all to see. Meeting other people offering a similar service to you will be beneficial rather than competition as you can learn from them and pick up tips and advice. Meeting and working with the general public will be extremely useful in knowing what people want and like.

The more you get out there working at what you love in whatever capacity you can, the more you will feel like the Reiki Practitioner you are aiming to be and people will become to see you as the Reiki Practitioner you are. As long as there is some sort of exchange of energy for the Reiki Treatment, it will be beneficial to you both. At first it may not be money at all, but a smile or a grateful hug. Friends may bake you a cake or treat you to a drink, but stick with it and the exchange of money will soon come.

As said before, swap treatments are a lovely way for practitioners of all different therapies, to exchange treatments with each other, enabling the importance of self care whilst meeting, networking and gaining more practise.

Self Reiki is great to give yourself each day if possible, but there is nothing like a full Reiki Treatment for yourself every now and again. I recommend it highly as it not only rebalances and restores your energy from top to toe but is also invaluable in working out how you wish to work as a Practitioner (and not!) The more you relax and get a taste of how other people work, the more you will become aware of your own tastes and your passion and therefore how you wish to work. We always have something to learn from every situation we are in and everyone we meet.

Beware of the Ego

Keep an eye on the ego as you progress and work with others. Reiki allows us to be a channel which we can use for self treatment and the treatment of others. When stepping into the role of Practitioner, it is an easy place to get confused as to what it is you exactly do. Our left brains and our ego need to have things to do constantly. They like us to feel very busy and very important but it's not like that with Reiki and this is something we must remind ourselves of regularly.

Reiki when practised as it should be, is very simple, a child can do it. We connect with the Universal Life Energy and through a series of hand positions, we act as a channel for this energy to flow through us whilst the recipient draws what they need. It is not for us to diagnose or prescribe any medical condition or treatment.

Also, it is not for the Practitioner to get so wrapped up in a client's situation that the lines of client/ practitioner get blurred. Understandably it is easy to get on well with clients especially if they become regular customers and there is nothing wrong with this, but a certain degree of detachment is necessary to enable you to conduct yourself professionally.

We must never presume that we know the best outcome for the client and we must remember that no amount of vested interest in them recovering from disease or illness will aid their recovery. Everyone is on his/her own path and one person's road along the way may be very very different to another's.

Don't take everything personally. If you see a client and then you never see them again, it doesn't mean you did anything wrong. One treatment may be all they needed. Sometimes people are surfing around trying different things and different places. Accept that not everyone will want to come to you and may prefer the Reiki Practitioner in the next street. Again, it is nothing personal - your energy just didn't fit with theirs, just as we don't all dress the same, or are attracted to the same people, activities, food, restaurants ....

Reiki practitioners work very differently from one person to the next. Some work intuitively, others with chakras, crystals, drums, tarot ... And many many more I'm sure. It is understandable that people will want to shop around to find the right fit for them. I list all these different ways that Reiki Practitioners may work, but obviously they are all practising Reiki, i.e. being a channel and putting their ego to one side but in their own unique way.

We don't take on the responsibility of everyone's well being either. You need to be present in the meeting you have with your client and do all that is required for a professional Reiki Treatment, but their health does not depend on you and you are in no way their salvation.

I like to think of everyone as being perfect but some may have a layer or two over their bright shining light, which needs help unravelling. However, it might be that the time is not right just yet for all the layers to come off just yet. Others may have many many layers built up over time and like peeling an onion, it is a slow but enjoyable journey seeing the protective layers being released.

Most caring professionals start out needing to be needed which is great, no-one wants a miserable person on autopilot as a Practitioner but that part of us needs to be monitored and that Ego needs keeping in check!

Top Tips For Being A Successful Reiki Practitioner

I am not going to list anything magical and mystical here, simply practical ways I have found to work to build up a practice and regular client base.

*   Create a safe, friendly, inviting and clean Treatment Room.
*   Make sure you are 'nice to be near' when practising Reiki.
*   Work out a pricing structure that you are happy with.
*   Give yourself plenty of time in between each Treatment.
*   Maintain your self care routine, however busy you get.
*   Keep records of everything.
*   Ground Yourself Regularly and step up your Self-Care routine.

Create a Safe, Friendly, Inviting and Clean Treatment Room

The World needs as many healers as possible! So find somewhere to practise and get practising! Just make it somewhere you would feel safe and nurtured in. People need a place to go to take respite from their life or day. Let them be as comfortable as possible with a comfortable bed, soft lighting and relaxing music. It doesn't need to cost you the earth. It needs to work for you and your family if you are working from home and your clients. If you have a spare room, I would advise, you start there, keeping your outlay to a minimum as you get established.

As I said earlier, I was literally in an under the stairs cupboard with no window, using a curtain as a room divider, but people loved it. I made it as welcoming as possible and my clients felt safe and calm. Garden rooms/summer houses, are very popular now. If you are lucky enough to have a garden, this is an excellent way of creating your own workspace. A nice distance away from the busy house, outside with nature and fairly inexpensive to build or buy.

The other alternative is to hire a room or share a room with another practitioner. Hairdressers often have rooms that they let out for treatments.

Make Sure You Are 'Nice To Be Near' When Practising Reiki

It is common sense but I must point it out. Who wants somebody with bad breath, body odour, rattling jewellery and hair all in their face, leaning all over them, whilst you try and relax for a Treatment. Think carefully about the clothes you choose to wear. I generally have 'work clothes' which are appropriate, freshly laundered and comfortable. Remember that odour clings to fabric, so try not to wear clothes you have been wearing whilst smoking if you smoke, or cooking in. Again, just present yourself how you would wish a Practitioner to greet you.

I was once met at the door when greeting a new client with the comment "Oh, I expected someone dressed all in purple with crystals in their hair!" I think there is an expectation of how maybe a Reiki Practitioner might look :-)

Work Out A Pricing Structure That You Are Happy With

It is very hard when first starting out. You know that you are newly trained and haven't much experience, so it seems hard to ask for anything at all. To be honest, you probably would be ecstatic to practise Reiki for free as you are so excited to be doing it all. However, as we are taught in our Reiki training, you have invested a lot of time and money in learning this new skill and now are in the position to share all you have learned with others. If you don't charge a fee, people would be uncomfortable in coming for a treatment and would definitely not feel they could ask to return. There needs to be an energy exchange for every service.

At first you may have started with volunteering and treating friends and family, but now you need to be professional. Do your market research and once you are informed, decide where you see yourself. Beware setting your price too low, as people may not perceive you to be confident and professional. Beware also setting your price too high, it needs to be in line with other services such as a massage treatment in you area. When deciding upon your pricing, bear in mind your location. Obviously prices in a large wealthy city, will bear no reflection on a small rural village location.

Think about your overheads, how much will it cost you to hire your treatment room, heat the room, replenish and maintain its upkeep. At the same time, exactly how much time are you spending on each treatment and how much is your hourly rate. Are you having to factor in child care costs?

Your business can only possibly be a success if it is financially viable and profitable. Your voluntary days are over, this is business now, you are giving people a great service and in this present age, it is very very much needed. So when people lie on your treatment bed remember, they are there for a reason and you are there to give service. The exchange is totally justifiable and there should be no difficulty for you taking your client's money in payment for the great service you are offering. Remember people are needing a great Reiki Practitioner and are happy to pay. So set your prices wherever your homework tells you they need to be and smile and confidently value your work.

Give Yourself Plenty of Time In Between Each Treatment

There may be times when everyone wants to come for a treatment on the same day at the same time! Beware, do not overstretch yourself. Book people in with plenty of time in between and don't go out of your way to be overly accommodating. You need to set some boundaries and decide when you wish to work and what suits you and your family. Maybe evenings and/or weekends would be a good place to start whilst you are able to work during the day at your existing job until you get enough clients. It is ok to let people know that you are busy and offer them an alternative appointment. If they want to come, they will come another day and respect that you have other clients to see.

You may not currently be aware of the logistics of running a practice, but you will need to prepare your room again for each client and ensure you are refreshed and notes written up. If you are standing mostly whilst practising, make sure you place a chair at the head and feet of the treatment table if possible which helps especially as these are areas you may be for longer periods.

Maintain Your Self Care Routine, However Busy You Get

Even if you have a busy day ahead, booked with clients, these are the days you must not let your self care routine slip. Practice your morning yoga routine, do your breathing exercises, stretch, eat breakfast, don't skip lunch, go for a walk, whatever it is that you need to do to be at your best.

You will know that you have not met this criteria if you feel at all unwell at the end of your day. A banging headache is a sure sign that you have not eaten or drunk enough or grounded yourself after each treatment. It does not mean that you cannot do this work or that you are taking on your clients problems and ailments, it just means that you need to work harder at looking after your 'self'. Remember you get Reiki as it comes through you, so this should help to keep you balanced to a certain extent.

Keep Records of Everything

When you set yourself up, keep all the receipts for all that you buy for your business. You will need to keep a record of clients, and the money you have made each year. You will need to devise a simple form to use during each visit with your clients and then keep these records for 7 years. Each visit with every client needs to be documented with how the treatment went and any resulting information. Little things like how many pillows people prefer, what music they like listening to and which blanket they always ask for can be noted so that you can refresh yourself prior to their visit and they will enjoy the personal attention to detail.

Ground Yourself Regularly

As an energy therapist, you are stepping into other people's energy constantly. Your auras are mingling and your energy will also be diminished a little whilst being busy and interacting with a variety of people. The Reiki is definitely coming through you and you will benefit to a certain degree, but don't depend on only this. Take steps to keep grounded.

When working with clients, your crown chakra is being opened up constantly and the energy is flooding in and through you. It can take it's toll and make you feel dizzy, weak, overloaded and scattered. If you are empathic your brow chakra will be opening up more and you may take on others' feelings for a moment on top of this, which you need to then offload. There are many techniques and you will need to find what works for you. Breathing, exercising, drinking plenty of water, (which you can Reiki prior to drinking), clearing your space, energising yourself with nature and getting outside, walking barefoot, eating natural food, meditating and exercising, are just a number of ways. It really is the total self care package.

Try to not book too much in one day, I would never see more than 4 people a day!

A Note About Being An Empath

I have to give all you empaths a mention here. If you've never heard of the word empath, don't worry, it just means that you probably are not one. However, please be aware, as a large amount of people drawn to Reiki seem to be on the empathic side.

A general definition of being an empath is someone with the strong ability to feel the thoughts, emotions and energy of others and generally are affected by these influences to the point of it becoming debilitating.

It is definitely possible to be a successful professional Reiki Practitioner and be empathic and in my view, I think it gives you the edge as you are literally tuning into your client whenever you practise Reiki. Your clients will love the connection you have with them. However, you will have to make your self care programme your number 1 priority over everything else! Otherwise you will not be able to sustain your practise for any length of time. As long as you look after yourself, you will be fine.

It will probably be best that you work in an environment that you have total control over, maybe from home. You will then be at ease and comfortable with the energy of the building and the room. If this is not possible, you can use space clearing techniques which we will go onto next and manage your energy levels in between each client carefully. I know of one lady practitioner who finds salt water very effective and has a little splash and freshen up after each client she sees.

Crystals are powerful and can act as a lifesaver and an empath's best friend. Wearing them as a necklace or in your pocket, to help shield, protect and preserve your energy.

The Reiki symbols are for your benefit when working with clients also, we mustn't forget this. The Power and Focus Symbol in particular is used for protection and can be used above you, beneath you and all around you, like an invisible cloak.

You could also imagine standing in the centre of a beautiful bubble or glass box, filled with whatever colour you need and see the top opening up and filling the entire space with Reiki Symbols.

I think the important advice to take here is to prepare yourself and your room prior to your client's treatment and then at the end of the treatment again. If during the treatment, you begin to feel unwell eg. a headache, or dizzy, you need to instantly recognise this and ground immediately. Open your eyes, take big, slow breaths, really feel the soles of your feet pressing down into the floor, wriggle your toes and if necessary, step away for a moment and have a drink of water. Then change your position and maybe sit at the head or feet instead.

You are in control of your own body and are separate from the person in front of you in a physical sense. As much as your energy may be merging with your client's, you maintain your separation with your mind. State before the treatment in your mind when you set your intention that you wish to be protected, you wish to maintain your own sense of physical separation from this person and that you do not wish to take on the client's emotions or physical ailments. If you have a connection with a spirit guide, spirit animal, gatekeeper, angel, archangel, ancestor .... call upon them every time you work and ask for their help and assistance.

Space Clearing

The space you work in is important, not only for your clients, as discussed before, but also for yourself. You need to feel the magic of the room and add to that magic each day. Your energy and love of the room will fill it up and all who enter will feel comfortable, nurtured and safe and not want to leave.

Initially, it is a good idea to clear the room by using your hands and your intention. Open a window, or door and as you walk around the room, get into all the corners, nooks and crannies, stating that you wish all lingering energy to leave and welcome in new positive fresh energy every day. You could use white sage and waft this around with a large feather or your hand, which is commonly used for clearing. Incense is a good alternative to sage. The smoke aids the clearing and is a visual tool to enable you to see where you are going and have been.

The 2nd Degree symbols can also be used for clearance and protection. Walk around the room, drawing symbols in the air, on the ceiling, floor and walls, saying their mantras three times, with the intention to clear the room, as described above. Don't forget under your Treatment Bed.
The symbols can also be drawn on the Treatment Bed and pillow, prior to your client arriving.

Crystals are powerful tools to use in raising energy and can be used with clients during Reiki but also within your room to aid the flow of energy and enhance energy levels. Crystals absorb energy, so placing above or near the doorway, will catch people's energy on entering and exiting. Placing them on windowsills and in the corners of the room are also great ways of directing energy.

Getting Organised

So, you've found your space, and made it beautiful and you're raring to go. It is a good idea to join a Reiki organisation or society when you are setting yourself up in business to practise. This is not only a great way for you to get professionally recognised but also helps you to be professionally consistent. You will be required to complete a certain amount of learning or research each year to renew your membership and I think it's a good healthy way of encouraging us to keep up to date. Your Reiki Master should be able to advise you about this and recommend an organisation or society to use.

Maintain professional standards by being organised. People need to be able to find you so make sure you are visible either via a website or on social media. I find this the biggest hurdle for most people. Even if social media is not your thing, to be busy with clients and regular work, it is something you need to embrace to reach the people and let them know what you are doing. I can assure you that you can retain your privacy, it is just your business face, your 'shop window' that needs to be visible. It may seem very alien and out of your comfort zone, but get some help, go on a course, quite often they are free, and get out there.

If you are going down the website route, a free template is all you need to start with. This can be done yourself at very little cost. You will need to pay for your domain name, which is your computer website name and address.

Obviously you will need to have thought of a name for yourself/your business. Again, this is a big sticking point for people. Brainstorm and check your ideas with others before committing. You don't want to spend on business cards etc. and then change your mind. If in doubt, your name is perfectly acceptable.

Should People Really Be Charging For Healing?

This title was to get your attention - Yes, Yes and Yes again! Absolutely they should. I don't understand why there are so many people struggling to make a living as Reiki Practitioners. The world really is an upside down place to be living in. We seem to de-value the people who are doing the greatest service to mankind and its planet. Our Firemen, Nurses, Lifeboat Rescue Teams, Ambulance Crews, Teachers, Nursery workers, Nursing Home Carers…. all get paid a pittance compared to other professions. There really needs to be a shift in the way we view our health and the health of our loved ones and those that care for them.

It starts with you and how you feel about the service you are providing. I urge you to please never forget all the time you have spent money training and all the experience you have gained with your daily self Reiki, self meditations, Reiki Shares and the Reiki you have been practising either on your friends and family or in the voluntary sector or charitable work.

Remember the sacrifices you have made and the enthusiasm you feel about doing this work. Get your self confidence and self worth in the place it needs to be before working with others. Heal yourself of any blocks or negativity that you may have around earning money and feeling worthwhile and deserving of every penny. Your clients need you to be totally confident and empowered in your work and they will feel this emanate from you and be more than happy to pay for your excellent confident service.

With belief, hard work and positivity, it really is absolutely possible to be doing something you love and get paid to do so.

Don't Analyse Things and Just Get Cracking!

I come across so many amazing people who are fantastic at practising Reiki and would be incredible Reiki Practitioners, but a very small percentage seem to go on to practise Reiki professionally. I think the main reason is, insecurity and so I try to offer as much support to my students as possible. I took forever to practise professionally myself and am lucky enough to have a very supportive husband, so I sympathise with this predicament.

I understand that Reiki is still a little niche, but in many ways this is it's advantage. If you can set yourself up, work hard and get known and get a good name for yourself, you have a niche business there, growing in popularity every day and getting more well known as each year passes. You will help to get Reiki out there and help to spread the word.

I also pick up that often students fear competition. This is so limiting and really just the mind putting problems in the way. There is no such thing as competition, only a community of support out there. Reiki Practitioners need each other and the more the merrier!
We often see cafes setting up next door to other cafes or antiques shops all nestling together in the same street. This is great for the customers as they get more choice and more people will be able to find them.

It will not generally be a quick start, as most of us start up as a hobby and do it 'on the side' but I think this allows for confidence to grow and us to get our hand in (excuse the pun). Most successful businesses start up in a spare room on a very small scale. I remember being thrilled with one client every now and again and just grateful and excited. I wasn't thinking about getting bigger or getting more clients, I just wanted to practise.

Enthusiasm gets you everywhere. If Reiki is something you love and just need to do, it's because you are meant to do it, so go for it! If you defer and defer until you are more ready, there may never be a time that you feel you are ready. I say, go for it and learn and grow each and every day. Every day, I feel that I am learning and feel that every client I meet has something to bring that I can learn from. Isn't that the beauty of life. When we know it all, it would surely become very boring.

What Sort of Practitioner Will You Be?

We are all offering something unique because of the life experience we bring with us. If you are unsure how to work with Reiki, just value who you are and list all your strengths and what you can bring with you to your Reiki business.

Are you good with people?
Do you have good business skills?
Are you coming from another profession that you could mix your Reiki skills with?
Do you have good organisation skills?
Are you good with paperwork?
Can you type?
Are you a good listener?
Are you empathic or highly sensitive?
Are you psychic?
Are you a good teacher?
Do you enjoy working on your own?
Do you enjoy working in a team?
Do you have good social media skills?
Do you have good marketing skills?
Are you good at maths?

Whatever your unique skills are, blend them together and use them to mould yourself into the best version of a Reiki Practitioner that works for you. If you are being yourself and doing what you love, others will also love who you are and what you do.

This is not an exhaustive list and I could go on. Basically every skill you possess will be helpful. When working for yourself, the learning curve is huge but comes in small steps, like climbing a ladder. Celebrate your strengths and realise that you may need help in areas you are not so confident about. Don't worry about your weaknesses: Celebrate your strengths. Don't let your fears prevent you from achieving your dreams.

Whatever you bring with you will determine how you practise and will make you totally unique.

There are so many ways Reiki can be practised and I find it really exciting. You never really know what to expect when you go for a Reiki Treatment and I think that's fabulous. It allows for freedom, diversity and creativity. Many practitioners are working with animals, plants, sound therapy, drumming, colour therapy, chakras, angels, light, tarot, crystals....

There are many different lineages of Reiki and each work with different symbols and techniques.

End Note

I really hope this book helps you to feel more confident about becoming a Reiki Practitioner. I know it can seem a big leap to make changes but by taking small steps each day, it can easily be achievable. Your limitation is only your imagination.

"Stay away from negative people, they have a problem for every solution"
Albert Einstein

Create a clear vision of your future and start taking action every day working towards it.

Good Luck!

Further information and contact;

stleonardsreiki.co.uk

stleonardsreiki@gmail.com

Facebook - St Leonards Reiki & EFT

Instagram - stleonardsreikiandeft

Printed in Great Britain
by Amazon

78222859R00048